The **Richard & Hinda Rosenthal Symposium**

2014

Antimicrobial Resistance:
A Problem Without Borders

INSTITUTE OF MEDICINE
OF THE NATIONAL ACADEMIES

THE NATIONAL ACADEMIES PRESS
Washington, D.C.
www.nap.edu

THE NATIONAL ACADEMIES PRESS • 500 Fifth Street, NW • Washington, DC 20001

NOTICE: The project that is the subject of this report was approved by the Governing Board of the National Research Council, whose members are drawn from the councils of the National Academy of Sciences, the National Academy of Engineering, and the Institute of Medicine.

Support for this project was provided by the Rosenthal Family Foundation.

International Standard Book Number-13: 978-0-309-31286-8
International Standard Book Number-10: 0-309-31286-8

Additional copies of this report are available from the National Academies Press, 500 Fifth Street, NW, Keck 360, Washington, DC 20001; (800) 624-6242 or (202) 334-3313; http://www.nap.edu.

For more information about the Institute of Medicine, visit the IOM home page at: **www.iom.edu.**

Suggested citation: IOM (Institute of Medicine). 2014. *The Richard & Hinda Rosenthal Symposium 2014: Antimicrobial Resistance: A Problem Without Borders.* Washington, DC: The National Academies Press.

"Knowing is not enough; we must apply.
Willing is not enough; we must do."
—Goethe

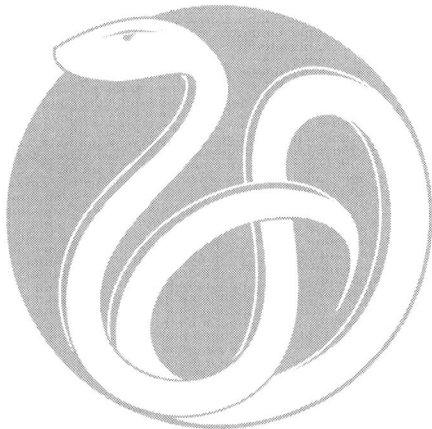

INSTITUTE OF MEDICINE
OF THE NATIONAL ACADEMIES

Advising the Nation. Improving Health.

THE NATIONAL ACADEMIES
Advisers to the Nation on Science, Engineering, and Medicine

The **National Academy of Sciences** is a private, nonprofit, self-perpetuating society of distinguished scholars engaged in scientific and engineering research, dedicated to the furtherance of science and technology and to their use for the general welfare. Upon the authority of the charter granted to it by the Congress in 1863, the Academy has a mandate that requires it to advise the federal government on scientific and technical matters. Dr. Ralph J. Cicerone is president of the National Academy of Sciences.

The **National Academy of Engineering** was established in 1964, under the charter of the National Academy of Sciences, as a parallel organization of outstanding engineers. It is autonomous in its administration and in the selection of its members, sharing with the National Academy of Sciences the responsibility for advising the federal government. The National Academy of Engineering also sponsors engineering programs aimed at meeting national needs, encourages education and research, and recognizes the superior achievements of engineers. Dr. C. D. Mote, Jr., is president of the National Academy of Engineering.

The **Institute of Medicine** was established in 1970 by the National Academy of Sciences to secure the services of eminent members of appropriate professions in the examination of policy matters pertaining to the health of the public. The Institute acts under the responsibility given to the National Academy of Sciences by its congressional charter to be an adviser to the federal government and, upon its own initiative, to identify issues of medical care, research, and education. Dr. Victor J. Dzau is president of the Institute of Medicine.

The **National Research Council** was organized by the National Academy of Sciences in 1916 to associate the broad community of science and technology with the Academy's purposes of furthering knowledge and advising the federal government. Functioning in accordance with general policies determined by the Academy, the Council has become the principal operating agency of both the National Academy of Sciences and the National Academy of Engineering in providing services to the government, the public, and the scientific and engineering communities. The Council is administered jointly by both Academies and the Institute of Medicine. Dr. Ralph J. Cicerone and Dr. C. D. Mote, Jr., are chair and vice chair, respectively, of the National Research Council.

www.national-academies.org

Foreword

The Institute of Medicine (IOM) launched an innovative outreach program in 1988. Through the generosity of the Rosenthal Family Foundation (formerly the Richard and Hinda Rosenthal Foundation), a discussion series was created to bring greater attention to some of the significant health policy issues facing our nation today. Each year a major health topic is addressed through remarks and conversation between experts in the field. The IOM later publishes the proceedings from this event for the benefit of a wider audience.

The Rosenthal events have attracted an enthusiastic following among health policy researchers and decision makers in Washington, DC, and across the country, and produce a dynamic and fruitful dialogue. In this volume, we are proud to present remarks by and an engaging discussion with Dr. Rima Khabbaz, Dr. Stuart Levy, Dr. Margaret (Peg) Riley, and Dr. Brad Spellberg on "Antimicrobial Resistance: A Problem Without Borders."

I would like to thank Daniel Bethea, Katharine Bothner, Leigh Carroll, Marton Cavani, Eileen Choffnes, Bradley Eckert, Greta Gorman, India Hook-Barnard, Patrick Kelley, Abbey Meltzer, Meghan Mott, Patsy Powell, Lauren Shern, and Liz Tyson for skillfully handling the many details associated with the symposium program and the publication.

In their lifetimes, Richard and Hinda Rosenthal accomplished a great deal. The annual Rosenthal Symposium at the IOM is among their enduring legacies, and we are privileged to be the steward of this important ongoing series.

Victor J. Dzau, M.D.
President
Institute of Medicine

Contents

Welcome

HARVEY V. FINEBERG

Good afternoon, everyone. I am Harvey Fineberg, President of the Institute of Medicine (IOM). It is my great pleasure to welcome all of you to this 2014 Richard & Hinda Rosenthal Symposium. Our topic this year is Antimicrobial Resistance: A Problem Without Borders.

This endowed lecture and symposium series is sponsored by the Rosenthal Family Foundation. It has been a special annual activity at the Institute of Medicine for more than a quarter century. Every year, we bring forward at these discussions a key health policy issue that is facing our country right now. We try to deal with that issue from a range of informed perspectives. The series has had many important leaders in health care and policy and academia, in government and in the private sector, who have participated.

The very first lecture in the Rosenthal series dealt with the question of providing universal and affordable health care. How little changes over time. Recently, we have had other symposiums that have dealt with important and critical topics, most recently last year, on the future of nursing, which was a very important subject for the Institute of Medicine, for the United States domestically, and, indeed, for the world.

Many of the subjects have really emphasized, particularly, the United States and our needs, in general, our health challenges. Today, we are going to be focusing on a topic that deals with every country in the world, truly a topic with global implications. As we will undoubtedly hear in the course of the presentations from our eminent panel, it requires global thought and collective action in order to find solutions.

Consider for a moment how much attention is now attending the problem of antimicrobial resistance. The Centers for Disease Control and Prevention (CDC) identified antimicrobial resistance as one of five urgent health threats facing the United States this year. In its recent report, *Antibiotic Resistance Threats in the United States*, released last year, the CDC notes that at least 2 million people in the United States acquire infections with bacteria that are resistant to one or more antibiotics and 23,000 deaths follow.

The White House launched, in its Global Health Security Agenda earlier this year, a recognition of the threat that is caused by the confluence of emerging microbes, globalization of food and travel, and increase in drug-resistant pathogens. The agenda at the White House calls for a diverse set of government agencies to work more closely together on these related problems, including the Department of Health and Human Services, especially the CDC, the Departments of Defense, of State, and of Agriculture, as well as USAID [U.S. Agency for International Development].

The World Health Organization (WHO) devoted its 2011 World Health Day to the topic of antimicrobial resistance, noting that many drug-resistant microbes render medications around the world ineffective and more will be ineffective in coming years. Last week, WHO released its first global report on antimicrobial resistance surveillance. Among the key findings that they released are, first, alarming increases in anti-microbial resistance and major gaps on the collection of surveillance data and the coordination of surveillance efforts. This report from WHO also described antimicrobial resistance as a global health security threat that will demand collaboration from many stakeholders around the world.

This is a topic that has been of sustained and important interest also here at the National Academies, at the National Research Council, especially in our Board on Life Sciences and our Division of Earth and Life Studies, and at the Institute of Medicine. It is of particular interest, for example, in the Institute of Medicine's Forum on Medical and Public Health Preparedness for Catastrophic Events. It has also had a direct bearing on the work of the Forum on Drug Discovery, Development, and Translation. Most especially, this topic has been central to the work of our Forum on Microbial Threats.

This forum was established in 1996 after the IOM published the report *Emerging Infections: Microbial Threats to Health in the United States*, which, in turn, followed a request from the CDC and the NIH [National Institutes of Health]. Initially, this forum was called the Forum on Emerging Infections, but the name was changed to Microbial Threats about a decade ago to reflect the more broad concerns. Many leaders in government, in academia, in industry, and from the public come together in this forum to illuminate ways that this field can be brought together and how we can more effectively deal with the problem of antimicrobial resistance. You will find as you leave if you have not noticed as you came in, a number of publications from the forum that you are welcome to take, including *Infectious Disease Movement in a Borderless World and Antibiotic Resistance: Implications for Global Health and Novel Intervention Strategies.*

In the course of our discussion this evening, we hope to highlight the crosscutting character of antimicrobial resistance and the needs for many disciplines to be brought together to be able to deal with it more effectively. It is not only a medical issue. It is not only a public health issue. It has significant implications for population well-being and security more broadly. It deserves to be a focus of attention for leaders in medicine, public health, agriculture, veterinary health, security, and policy more broadly.

We have a very, very distinguished panel with us tonight. I am very pleased to be able to introduce them to you. As I do, I also want to take just a moment to acknowledge and to thank the staff who have made this evening possible. First, I want to thank Lauren Shern and Brad Eckert for organizing this event. Thank you both so very, very much. I also want to acknowledge the leadership of Clyde Behney, our Interim Leonard D. Schaeffer Executive Officer at the Institute of Medicine, who has overseen the development of tonight's event, and to thank Meghan Mott at registration, who has been helping us this evening, particularly, to make all of our entries so smooth.

Now, to introduce the four panelists, I am going to introduce them in the reverse order that they will be speaking. The last will be introduced first. At the end, I will introduce the first of the speakers.

The speaker who will come toward the end is Dr. Brad Spellberg. Brad is Associate Medical Director for Inpatient Services and Associate Program Director for the Internal Medicine Residency Training Program at the Harbor-UCLA Medical Center. His work with the Infectious Disease Society of America and particularly a number of position papers that he has put forward based on a dataset related to new drug development has certainly raised considerable attention to the problem of antimicrobial resistance. Indeed, it is going to be a pleasure for us to hear Brad's comments this evening.

Just before Brad speaks, Dr. Peg Riley will address us. Peg Riley is a Professor in the Department of Biology at the University of Massachusetts Amherst. Her research focuses on, among other things, the evolution of antibiotic resistance and the development of novel antimicrobials. Dr. Riley was a member of the National Research Council's Committee on New Directions in the Study of Antimicrobial Therapeutics and currently serves as a member of the NRC's Board on Life Sciences. Thank you so very much for being with us tonight.

Our second speaker will be Dr. Stuart Levy. Dr. Levy is Distinguished Professor of Molecular Biology and Microbiology and of Medicine and Director of the Center for Adaptation Genetics and Drug Resistance at Tufts University Medical School. He is also the cofounder and the president of the Alliance for the Prudent Use of Antibiotics. This organization, established in 1981, conducts public health advocacy, research, and surveillance, as well as consumer and practitioner engagement and education. It has, over the years, developed more than 60 affiliated chapters around the globe, an important institutional achievement. It will be a pleasure, Stuart, to hear from you.

Our first speaker this evening, Dr. Rima Khabbaz, is the Deputy Director of Infectious Diseases and Director of the Office of Infectious Diseases at the CDC. Dr. Khabbaz has held positions at the CDC since 1980, beginning as an epidemic intelligence service officer in the National Center for Infectious Diseases' Hospital Infections Program. She has seen this problem in virtually every expression and in every setting over the years. I am very grateful to Rima, also, for her service as a member of the Institute of Medicine's Forum on Microbial Threats.

More complete background information on some of the achievements and experience of our speakers may be found in the program. I know you will enjoy as much as I hearing from each and then participating in the roundtable discussion that will follow. Now, let me turn to Rima Khabbaz, our first speaker. The floor is yours.

Panelist Remarks and Discussion

DR. KHABBAZ: Thank you very much. Thank you very much, both for the introduction and the opportunity to participate on this panel. Obviously, to me, the topic of antimicrobial resistance is dear to my heart because I have dealt with it, as Harvey said, for many, many years. It is rewarding to finally see it getting the attention that it deserves.

It is a major, major public health problem and one of our most serious health threats, no question. I know we are talking about antimicrobial resistance, but really the urgency and the need for immediate action is really for antibacterial resistance. I will touch on why. Not that the resistance across the board with viruses and specific microbes is not important, it is very important, but the urgency is really with antibacterial agents.

At CDC, where I work, we have three strategic directions that my boss, Director Tom Frieden, has articulated for us to focus our work. I mention them, keep in mind, because antibiotic resistance touches on all three. One is health security. Dr. Fineberg mentioned the antimicrobial threat as really a concern, a priority health threat here, domestically, and around the world. The CDC report estimated 2 million illnesses caused by antibiotic resistance—that is probably an underestimate given the limitation of our data—and 23,000 deaths, and associated costs of up to maybe $20 billion is excess direct health care costs from antibiotic resistance.

Globally, the WHO report on resistance echoes the concerns and how antibacterial resistance touches every country and every region. It is serious. There is also a problem with lack of knowledge, inadequate knowledge, and inadequate surveillance systems to address it. So, health security.

Second is better preventing leading causes of death; preventing illnesses and death is obviously a focus.

Third is the need to strengthen public health and health care collaboration on antibiotic resistance to deal with the problem. Really, this is where it comes together. Both the health care system and health care providers, we feel, are at the center of the action that we can take now to slow the trends and really reverse them, both in terms of strengthening infection prevention in health care facilities and prevention interventions in communities, and then stewardship.

One of the, actually, *the* main driver for antibiotic resistance is use. Dr. Levy can probably say more and more elegantly than I about how this is not a new problem. The more we use antibiotics, the more the bacteria get smarter and fight back and develop resistance. We use a lot of antibiotics. We have a study that has shown that just in human health care, 30 to 50 percent of antibiotics that are prescribed to people here in the United States, are either not needed, don't need to get them, or they are prescribed inappropriately, for example in the wrong doses. There is a lot of that. Then in the veterinary/agricultural practice there is also a lot of antibiotic use and a lot of it is not for treatment and prevention. That is the main driver.

The confluence of drivers that have accelerated and elevated the concern is all of this use. Of course, contributing as well is globalization and people moving. The forms of resistance are very quickly, more quickly than ever, moving across international borders. Sometimes they arise somewhere and we detect them elsewhere.

Third, of course, is the fact that we do not have and we are not making any new antibiotic drugs. We haven't had them. This idea of continuing to make new ones that are more powerful seems to have ended.

There is a cost if we don't do anything. I mentioned the health care costs, but that is really moderate compared to what we are dealing with. The cost of inaction is huge and unimaginable. It almost kind of sounds like a doomsday scenario, but it is real. People talk about returning to a pre-antibiotic era where simple infections, say a cut of a finger, cannot be treated. That is real. We have some pathogens where we no longer have any antibiotic that fights them. There have been some stories and documentaries that have shown that with faces and people. It is real. It is here. It is with us.

Modern medicine as we know it with all of the joint replacement, knee and hip replacement, transplants, chemotherapy, dialysis, and other surgical procedures is predicated and dependent on antibiotics and our ability to treat and prevent infections. That goes away and we are in trouble. Everything becomes riskier. It is serious.

Now, there are things, like I said, that we can do to slow the tide. The CDC fiscal year 2015 budget request has $30 million so we can start implementing some strategic programs to strategically slow down and reverse the trends. The report [*Antibiotic Resistance Threats in the United States*] that Dr. Fineberg mentioned actually highlights the core actions that we feel are necessary.

A focus on prevention has also been mentioned. Prevention is core. It is basic, but if you prevent infection, you prevent the spread of resistance, and so that needs to happen. More of it needs to happen. There are some specific activities and collaboratives around that, as well as improving stewardship programs in hospitals. Every hospital should have a stewardship program. There are really things for everyone in a health care facility to do. Stewardship also goes beyond health care and hospitals.

Basically, improving the way we use antibiotics is important. Targeted prevention and antibiotic use—both of these have shown in studies and actually in examples where they really work. With MRSA, methicillin-resistant *Staphylococcus aureus*, for example, we have seen trends go down for invasive, serious MRSA based on those two pillars here.

Of course, we need to also improve our ability to detect and track antibiotic resistance. We have new technologies, molecular tools and genomic-based tools, which can really make a huge difference. New diagnostic tests can allow us to track resistance transmission better.

Finally, we do have some new, innovative thought, and are finding new ways to really accelerate the development of drugs and identifying new ways to stop this cycle. That is going to need concerted action and public–private partnerships.

The good news is that it is finally getting a lot of attention. Certainly, there is much interest in Congress in antibiotic resistance, also in the White House, as mentioned by Dr. Fineberg. The President's Council of Advisors on Science and Technology is preparing a major report. There are a lot of other activities and collaborations here across federal agencies and others and with other partners, as well as internationally with our European colleagues. A Transatlantic Taskforce on Antimicrobial Resistance, headed by HHS, has been focused on promoting collaborations and learning from each other. They will be coming up with a report on that soon.

WHO, as well, is very, very concerned and has reached across sectors to animal health and other sectors as well, and has formed a strategic and technical advisory group that I serve on. They are enthusiastic about action and are taking to the World Health Assembly in a couple of weeks a resolution to charge them with developing a global action plan that then can translate into regional and country action plans. It is one that they will lead and catalyze. It is not something that they can do alone. Like I said, it is a cross-sectoral thing.

I think it is a very serious problem, but one that we can do something about. Hopefully, with the interest and realization of how bad it is, maybe we can start turning the tide. Thank you.

DR. LEVY: Good evening, everybody. I thank the organizers for including me. I think Rima's remarks were very appropriate in the sense that there is an urgency. Some of you have been with me on a road that just seems to keep going on and on without an ending. I think maybe now we will see some changes. We see the White House getting involved. We see legislature getting more involved. I tell my students: science just goes so far, but after that, you need money and you need support from the government. I am hoping that is something we will get.

I really have not put together a formal talk so I will just tell you what I am thinking. First, let's go to the bacterium and then I will go to people and maybe go back to the bacterium. The point is if you are a bacterium and you are confronted by antibiotics, what do you do? You don't just gasp. You start making more bacteria, but these are resistant to the antibiotic.

The bacterium has only one thing to do in life: live, survive. We [humans] have lots of complications. They are simple. They have one chromosome. They have trouble with this on a daily basis, especially with us, who are trying to destroy them. Quite honestly, our newest goal is not to destroy them, but to bring them in and, like the new discoveries with the microbiomes, use the bacteria as our allies in shaping the world and keeping resistance in control.

How do bacteria become resistant? They acquire resistance genes. I will not talk down to you about the story, but it is a fascinating genetics story. I was doing work in France when I heard a talk on infectious antibiotic resistance. A Japanese co-worker, who worked with Tsutomu Watanabe, who I had the pleasure to work with—one of the forefathers of this field—was explaining that, in fact, the genes for resistance antibiotics were being transferred to other bacteria.

Joshua Lederberg found episomes going back and forth, but nobody had seen what they were seeing, which is, one or four different antibiotic resistances being transferred, and that they were transferred between a *Salmonella* and an *E. coli*. Then, as more and more data came out, more transferable resistances were being found, hence, infectious disease and infectious antibiotic resistance. That is a concept that I think you have to keep in mind because bacteria are always trying to get ahead of us. It is not as if I am giving them a brain, but at least they have residual energy to be able to survive.

The genetics are fascinating. I always thought of them as sort of science fiction. In the days before this kind of resistance was here, we would hear about bacterium moving four different resistances from one to another. Wow. I remember the first gels that Stan Falkow [Robert W. and Vivian K. Cahill Professor in Cancer Research, Emeritus, Stanford University School of Medicine] did showing that this was an episome or a piece of DNA that is transferrable.

I guess now would be a moment to try to let all of you who are not geneticists know that the genetics are fascinating. We have lots of names for them. We have plasmids. We have integrons. We have transposons. We have all these names because there is a variety of genetic mechanisms by which bacteria transfer resistances to others in the environment. The critical feature I want to stress is that their transfer of DNA is to different bacteria that are evolutionarily more diverse than a dog and a cat. That is a unique feature. That is what we began to see and began to face. Put that on the blackboard to say we have to deal with that at some point.

The other area has to do with the global feature of resistance. In 1981, we had a meeting in the Dominican Republic to which we brought several hundred people. It was the first time that a meeting outside the United States was sponsored by the NIH. Who was there? There were South Americans, Asians, all bringing their unusual resistance genes or resistant bacteria. Among those who were there, also, were sophisticated geneticists and microbiologists who were using these to discover new antibiotic resistances and all the fame and glory associated. What was curious was that the discoverers were not really, previously, part of the process of finding out what is going on. That meeting, I think, changed things. It established relationships between individuals in different countries, but not relationships where researchers would say, "I found this unusual resistance and I am going to give it to this French person or this American to work on."

Why and how do bacteria resist? They destroy the antibiotic. They don't let it get inside the cell because they pump it out. They substitute it with a new target, which is not subject to the resistance. There are very many different ways in which the bacteria escape the action of the antibiotic. That is also important to realize because that gives them a greater ability to escape.

The other feature of resistance that I think has not been shared largely is the enormous spread that resistance can take. In that regard, where do these resistances come from? I am asked that all the time. I say go out in your backyard and just grab some of the soil and you will find it. In fact, we coined this term "reservoirs of antibiotic resistance," which could be your backyard or someone's sandbox.

There is a huge quantity of bacteria out there with resistance genes that we don't even know about. They are waiting for an antibiotic to come on board so they can be expressed. In fact, that is how it happens, isn't it? What I call the antibiotic resistance equation requires two basic features. One is the antibiotic. And, two, if there are not resistance genes around, the antibiotic does its job. It is not resisted. It does fine. On the other hand, if the resistance gene gets into the mix, now, what you have is a resistant-bacterium and eventually a resistant infection. Resistance then takes over. It is an interesting phenomenon on how you can develop resistance slowly. But, essentially, in my mind, you need the gene or genes for resistance and you need the antibiotic to set the stage.

There is a lot of talk about what is going on in the animal world in terms of giving antibiotics. I think the One Health idea is really fascinating and best displayed in our field of antibiotic resistance. These bacteria have a link—there is a link between people and nature and veterinarians and the world. That connection is often through people or through the bacteria, themselves. There is a lot of discussion on the fate of the antibiotics that are being given to animals for animal health and, more so, for growth promotion.

It is an area that we, at the Center for Adaptation Genetics and Drug Resistance, have been looking at for years, and an argument that I have been working on with the FDA for years. Nothing has happened. Europe has banned this practice, but the United States continues. There is more activity coming aboard, more resentment, more pleas to change things, but Europe doesn't have it and we still do. I can only hope that will change.

What is the fate of the antibiotics given to animals? Well, they are distributed in nature. Looking at something simple like tetracycline, which is given to chickens and given to cattle and so forth—what happens with the antibiotic? It gets spread into the farm. It rains. The rain water takes the antibiotic down into the ground into other waterways and disperses it widely. Does anyone follow it? Not really. Does anyone know about it? Not really, or at least not in the way of understanding how this happens, but the phenomenon exists.

The second part of that, and something that I hear often is, well, you are treating and giving these animals low doses—that is important—of tetracycline. The resistances that you are claiming are coming from animals are to ampicillin and to aminoglycosides and others. How can that arise from the dosing of animals with one antibiotic?

Well, Naomi Datta gave us a hint about that many years ago. She looked at the antibiotic resistance profile of women taking antibiotics for urinary tract infections. Where did she look? Not in the urine, but in the feces. What she found was with time, instead of just one resistance, the women were accumulating different resistances. Where and how? On these plasmids, these genetic elements that bacteria have and that move resistances back and forth. That is an important concept because we are confronted with the thought of what happens after the antibiotic sees the animal group.

The studies we have done on farms and what other farms have shown that the use of a single antibiotic for 7 to 10 days will lead to an emergence of resistance to that antibiotic, but at 7, 8, 9, or 10 days, you suddenly see other resistances emerge. Fascinating. Where do they come from? Well, no one really knows, but some investigators in France had an idea. They saw that the chickens they were feeding antibiotic-laced feed were doing fine, but eventually were excreting resistant-bacteria, not just to tetracycline, but to other antibiotics. They sat back and they looked at the chickens for a while. This is a true story. They saw that the chickens didn't stop eating. When they went to look for the mystery resistances they took a gram of feed and they shook it up with a medium and they plated it. They didn't get the antibiotic-resistant bacterium. When they looked at these chickens merrily eating the feed, they realized they didn't stop at one gram. They went on to two grams, three grams worth. The next time they did the experiment, they took 10 grams of feed. They extracted the resistant bacteria.

It is in the design of the experiment how you can really find the answers. This was a very simple experiment, but it opened up, in my mind, the ideas of what was needed in order to confront arguments in the area of antibiotic supplementation.

Thank you very much.

DR. RILEY: It is always a pleasure to follow Stuart because he gets you to think from the perspective of microbial ecologists and that is what I am. I study the ecology of bacteria, and in particular, the evolutionary history of the resistance genes they carry.

Now, I am a little out of place here because in my lab, we are focused on the microbes. Here, all I see is a bunch of humans. I was told I can't use PowerPoints, but nobody told me I couldn't bring props. I brought my microbiome. What is wonderful about my microbiome is it is beautiful, it is colorful and diverse, and it is mine. It is not yours, Stuart. You have your own. This is my microbiome.

Each of you has a microbiome. That is the reason or part of the reason you are healthy, that you grow to your full potential, that you can consume the foods you want and get nutrition out of them. It is these guys doing their job.

What I would like to do is tell you a story. I went to a doctor once. A lot of women in the audience have had a urinary tract infection (UTI), I am sure. Often, 80 percent of the time, in community-acquired UTIs, the culprit is an *E. coli*. I went to the doctor and said, "Here are the symptoms. What are we going to do?" My doctor, very progressive, said, "I am not going to bother taking a culture. It is probably *E. coli*. Take this antibiotic. Go home. Do the full course, Peg, because we don't want resistance growing."

What do I do? I go home and I take this antibiotic. It is like the equivalent of an H-bomb for my microbiome. All of my microbes get decimated. Why do I say that? Nine out of every 10 cells in my body is a microbe. I am going to say that again because some people are surprised still: 9 out of every 10 cells in this body are these microbes that are making me healthy. When we use conventional antibiotics, we are essentially using what is analogous to a hydrogen bomb. We are just decimating the majority of our body's cells, which are microbial.

Now, certainly, some will survive. In my case, my *E. coli* survived because it was resistant. When we don't culture the bugs and test them for sensitivity to antibiotics, we will often misuse drugs and be given the wrong drug.

I am an experimentalist, so I gathered up my microbiome. My friend said, "Peg, eat yogurt, take probiotics. You microbiome will come back."

So, I have it back now. I got my microbiome back, including my *E. coli*. This time I did what I should have done the first time as a microbial ecologist. I should have said to my microbes, "Hey, microbes, I have a problem and I would like you to solve it for me. Would you?" As quick as that, the problem was gone.

What did they do? There was no H-bomb involved. It was one other bacterium, who happened to be a very close relative to that nasty one, the *E. coli*, which is now dead. This other bacterium produced a protein that specifically targeted my urinary tract infection strain, but no other microbes. In fact, the rest of the microbiome was having a party and didn't realize this little battle was being waged. They had no idea because this guy did its job right.

Now, why does that make sense? Because bacteria do not live in isolation. They can't live in isolation. They need this consort, this diverse community to make a living.

Let's compare and contrast the two views. We have utilized the fact that a very few lineages of bacteria produce conventional, broad-spectrum antibiotics: penicillin, ampicillin, tigecyclines. When we use them it is the equivalent of an H-bomb and the outcomes are pretty bad. First, they often don't work anymore. That is why we are all here. Second, they actually cause problems *to* us. Our body responds in negative ways. We get things like oral thrush or diarrhea. We feel pretty bad. Third, they select for intensely high levels of resistance. If my microbiome is, and I am just going to guess, 10^{18} cells and the mutation rate to the resistance is 10^{-6}, you do the math. I already have thousands of resistant strains in my body just through spontaneous mutations. This is not a good thing.

Now, let's look at what the microbes have done over 2.5 billion years. They have invented a different approach; it is called the guided missile. You remember watching CNN during the Gulf War, and all of a sudden we had these views of the guided missile going right down into a building in the middle of downtown Baghdad. The guided missile is the way microbes have evolved to deal with the interactions that go astray in their communities. They don't decimate their communities. That is just a foolish thing for them to do. They have evolved this sophisticated defense system that includes things like bacteriocins, which I would imagine some of you have never heard of, but you will in the next 15 years, and phage. Many of you have heard of phage. Those things are pretty powerful as a defense system. *E. coli* can kill other *E. coli* with a phage. *E. coli* can kill other *E. coli* with a bacteriocin.

I just want us to think for a minute about these two approaches. The first approach is what pharmaceutical industries have been prodded to do. We keep asking them to develop more antibiotics. We need them. We are desperate. We are dying. Their business model is based on a single pill that does the job. I think it was Albert Einstein who said if you do the same thing over and over again and expect a different result, that is the definition of insanity. We are asking the pharmaceutical companies to essentially be insane, because we know the outcome: another tigecycline, another chloramphenicol, another penicillin will simply select for massive resistance as soon as it is on the market. That is exactly what has happened with the very few novel antibiotics we have produced in the last few years.

We need to refocus our energies on this problem in several ways. First, we have to regard the microbiome. They are precious to us. They deserve and we owe them our respect. They deserve our respect because they are what make us feel good, feel healthy, and function properly.

Second, they are far wiser than we are. They have seen it all in 2.5 billion years. If you think you are going to invent a new drug that they can't resist, well, I am really sorry, but that is just silly. They have already got it. As Stuart was talking about, there are genes out there that have nothing to do with antibiotics that they will co-opt in half a second. If they are going to try to survive in the face of that drug, they will find a way to do it.

Finally, why not learn from these microbes? We have a plethora of new drugs to look at, to explore, to begin to imagine whether they might serve as the new paradigm in "attacking" infectious disease. I use that word in humor because we shouldn't be attacking anything. These are misunderstandings that are happening in our bodies, and we have to figure out ways to get rid of the misunderstandings.

One approach I have done in the last 15 years is—because I couldn't get the pharmaceutical industry involved—I started a small company on my own. We are about to release a drug to the veterinary community that will deal with mastitis. How will they do it? With exactly the same molecule that I used to kill that UTI strain. No collateral damage. No strong selection for resistance. Best of all, it works. It is not toxic. You have probably eaten that drug on foods in McDonald's if you have ever gone to the salad bar. Your body doesn't recognize it as a problem.

That is just one possibility amongst the many that exist that the basic biologists and microbiologists are exploring. Our job, now, should be to say, "We need something new. Let's try something different." Above all, let's love our microbiomes. Thank you.

DR. SPELLBERG: That is a great transition point because I think one of the central messages Peg has left us with is that what we are doing now is not working. We know it is not working because here we are talking about how bad things are, despite everything that we are doing. If we want to have a future state where we are not living with a crisis of antibiotic resistance, we need to think disruptively. Incrementally tweaking what we are doing is not going to get the job done. As we think disruptively and transformationally, to me, there needs to be a central core principle that I fear we have not paid attention to in policy or regulations that deal with antibiotics.

That core principle is that antibiotics are different than all other classes of drugs because only antibiotics suffer from transmissible loss of efficacy over time. That distinguishes them from all other classes of drugs. If you try to lump antibiotics in with other classes of drugs from a policy or regulatory perspective, you are going to focus on the wrong things and you are going to actually cause damage. I will give you some examples of that in a few moments.

From that core principle, I am going to talk about three areas that I would like to see transformation in. First, we need to do a much better job of protecting the antibiotics that we already have. Several speakers have mentioned antibiotics in animal feed. This is a national disgrace. There is no scientific debate here. I am not going to belabor this point. It needs to end. This is a political concern. When we get the political will, it will end. I am not going to say anything more about that now. We can talk more about it during the question and answer period.

More challenging to think about, scientifically, is how we prevent inappropriate antibiotic prescriptions among people. The traditional stewardship efforts—stewardship being the term we use to focus on giving the right antibiotic to the right people and not giving it when not necessary—relate to education, what I would call nagging, and local restriction efforts. These are important things to continue doing, but they only scratch the surface of the problem. This is putting a Band-Aid on the problem. This does not get to the root cause of why inappropriate prescriptions occur. If you want to deal with the root problem of why do they occur, it is simply fear. It is fear of the unknown. We, as treating physicians, do not, in fact, know what our patients have with certainty. We make our best guess. That guess is haunted by the fear that we could be wrong. That is what leads to physicians saying, "What if it is bacterial? How much harm could one prescription do?" It is the classic tragedy of the commons. If you want to combat the tragedy of the commons in this circumstance, you have to deal with that fear. Everything else is putting a Band-Aid on the problem.

How do we deal with that fear? Rapid diagnostics. We need technology. Relying upon asking people to behave differently in a sustainable way is not going to get the job done. That is the hardest thing to do in quality management. Technology can embed change. The technologies for rapid diagnostics are becoming available. We need regulators and payers, especially payers, to help us push these technologies into the clinic so that doctors don't have the fear that causes the inappropriate antibiotic prescription. We need to hold health care systems accountable for implementing these technologies as they become available.

We also need to harness the power of economics. I would like to see public reporting of antibiotic use across health care systems so that we can implement pay-for-performance metrics. Systems in the lowest quartile of use will get a payment bonus. Systems in the highest quartile of use will get a payment penalty. This strategy has been highly effective at driving down hospital-acquired adverse event rates of a variety of types. We need to seriously consider doing this, as well, because it will help us drive down overall antibiotic usage rates in patients.

Now, what is most disruptive, and where we are going to run into the most difficulties at a regulatory level and in industry, is recognizing that how we label antibiotics has to change. The way we label antibiotics, unfortunately, accidentally encourages inappropriate antibiotic pre-scriptions. As we have said, antibiotics are kind of a community property because of this transmissible loss of efficacy. Every individual's use of an antibiotic affects the ability of everybody else to use those antibiotics.

Take, for example, a broad-spectrum antibiotic that can kill Gram-negative pathogens that are highly resistant that I need because I don't have alternatives. It also kills staph and strep, which I have 20 other drugs to treat, and so I give an indication to that drug to treat staph and strep skin infections. Once that drug has that indication, the companies can market it for that indication. Like with all other drugs, marketing is what drives physician use of antibiotics. Now, the company is marketing the drug to, and the vast majority of its use is to, treat common staphylococcal and streptococcal infections that I have many other options to treat. I am selecting resistance to the drug. I can no longer use it to treat the Gram-negatives, which is what it is really needed for.

We need to consider appropriate antibiotic use when we label antibiotics. That is different than how the Food and Drug Administration (FDA) labels all other drug types. There is no precedent for doing this with drugs. I have already told you the core principle, which is that antibiotics are different than all other drug types. We need to recognize that in policy.

It may well be that the FDA doesn't have the statutory authority to consider appropriate use when it labels antibiotics. If that is the case, then we need to go to Congress and get that authority, but we should begin a dialogue with the FDA to find out what they could do with current regulations and what the gap is so we can talk to Congress about filling it.

Let me move on to discuss the antibiotic pipeline. How are we going to rekindle the pipeline? Because we absolutely do need new antibiotics. They are the most effective medications that we have in our pharmacopeia. We have economic challenges—antibiotics are a bad investment vehicle for companies—and we have regulatory challenges.

I am not going to talk about individual incentives because I don't have time. What I am going to say is that the traditional entrepreneurial business model for pharmaceutical companies to develop drugs does not work anymore for antibiotics. It is broken. In the future, we are going to need to move much more to a public–private partnership model. Some companies are leading the way. GlaxoSmithKline, for example, and Achaogen are already doing this. This is the future of antibiotic development in industry, public–private partnerships, defraying upfront cost and risk, and allowing the public a much bigger say into which drugs will get developed so that the market stops getting flooded with new skin drugs that we don't need any more of and start getting drugs to treat infections we are running out of drugs to treat.

This will require new regulatory pathways. If you are going to focus on unmet need, that is not something industry has done in the past. We are going to need new regulatory pathways to make that possible. We also need to continue the current efforts that are under way to reform traditional pathways. Right now, it is very difficult to enroll patients in antibiotic trials in the United States. That has to change.

Finally, I would like to echo thoughts that Peg introduced. All of our efforts to treat infections focus on killing the bug. It is incredibly effective as a therapeutic. It saves lives to a degree that other drugs simply can't match. It also drives resistance.

It is time for us, scientifically, to begin to transform, not to replace, antibiotics—to complement them, to take the pressure off them. Why do we have to kill the bug? This is a notion that dates back to a classic paper in the *Lancet* from Paul Ehrlich in 1913. You can trace the roots of the "to treat infection, kill the bug" approach to this 1913 article. Maybe we don't have to kill the bug. Maybe we can disarm the bug so that it doesn't cause disease, even if it is present, without trying to kill it.

Maybe we can passively starve it of nutrients that it has to get from the host in order to grow, or use probiotics to outcompete it, or not worry about the bug at all. Maybe we need to modulate the host inflammatory response. The signs and symptoms of infections that we experience as clinical disease are driven in many infections much more so by the host response to the bacteria than by any specific activity that the bacteria undertakes in our body. We can directly target host proteins and modulate that inflammatory response. All of these approaches will have much less propensity to select for resistance because we are not trying to kill the bug.

Scientifically, we need increased funding in this area. From a regulatory perspective, these new types of therapies are going to need new clinical development programs. They are not going to be developed in the traditional way that antibiotics are developed. Finally, we need to make sure new therapies are considered antibacterials so they can access legislative incentives that currently are focused on antibiotics that kill the bug. Thank you.

DR. FINEBERG: Thank you so much, Brad. Thank you all for a really fascinating set of introductory comments. The title for the session was *A Problem Without Borders*. I think we have to wonder is it also a problem without end? We had a number of allusions to ideas that could make a positive difference. We talked briefly about agricultural use of antibiotics. We talked about the overuse and misuse of existing antimicrobials. We talked about strategies for novel interventions, which are different from the conventional antimicrobial.

My basic question to you is what do you think is the avenue that we can pursue that will actually make this a problem one of history and not of the future? Is there a strategy that could work? Are all of these just stopgaps against an inevitable evolutionary force where bacteria are going to do what they need to do to survive, to use us as well as everything else for their nutrient needs, and to be ultimately successful? What is the mix of actions that are going to make the difference?

DR. KHABBAZ: It is a very complex problem. I think, all of the above. There are some things that we can and should do to slow the problem and protect existing drugs and prolong their effectiveness. That is something that is alluded to in the CDC's Detect and Protect Against Antibiotic Resistance initiative, where, clearly, we have examples of successes with CRE [carbapeneum-resistant Enterobacteriaceae] and MRSA [methicillin-resistant *Staphylococcus aureus*]. You get on top of antibiotic use, you do prevention—focused infection prevention—and you can make a difference. That is the immediate effort here.

As Brad said, we need new and better diagnostics so that physicians and health care providers can target the treatment more specifically and effectively. We need stewardship, as well. There is no question. I mentioned that 30 to 50 percent of antibiotics are prescribed with no indication or inappropriately. We have rates of antibiotic use across health care, across hospitals, that vary three times. Yes, there is an issue of physicians not knowing what they are treating, but there are also patients that get started on an antibiotic and then forget what they are on, so stewardship programs are important. We are working with the American Hospital Association and others on this. There are clearly some systematic approaches that can be taken at all levels of the health care system. We need to better track and identify new resistance so we can control it better.

As my co-panelists mentioned, the microbiome is really changing our paradigm of thinking, in terms of new approaches that we need to deal with bacteria. There are approaches we can use now and there are some we can use longer term. There is a challenge with clinical trials. NIH is thinking about it and thinking of a broader clinical trial network. In our budget initiative, we talk about networks—lab networks associated with a resistant bacteria bank—that will help us speed identification of these resistances, characterize them better, and make them available for the research that is needed, in terms of drugs and in terms of diagnostics and in terms of newer ways of dealing with infection.

DR. FINEBERG: Thank you, Rima. Do others want to comment? What mix of strategies do you think will make the difference in this? Stuart, why don't you go next?

DR. LEVY: I think one has to think about the organism and the infection at the same time. Brad was talking about antibiotics being unusual. I have always called them societal drugs because one person's use affects the rest of society. I think one can, similarly, now add to that the microbiome. If we are going to talk about doing something, maybe we should be thinking about how the microbiome could work for us, in which case, we come back to what we all have learned in medical school and elsewhere—that bacteria don't live in a vacuum and they aren't by themselves in any of the infections or any of the physiologies. We have to think of them as partners in a world that is microbial. We have to realize that this is a microbial world that we are currently in.

I think that refreshing and new looks at approaches, both immediate and prolonged, are needed. It would be great if we could develop novel approaches to infectious diseases, one of which we are actually practicing, which is to prevent the infection in the first place. You know there is going to be an infection so you treat with a nonantibiotic, which prevents the organism from pulling its machinery around to survive. It just never gets to make an infection.

I think what I am trying to do is put it together as a plurality, where you have bacteria, people, and governments involved. Each of them has a different role to play, but it is not one role. I think that what we have been talking about here is if we use killing of the bacterium as the end-all, then we are going to continue to propagate what we are in now.

DR. FINEBERG: Let me pick up on that because, actually, Peg, both you and Brad talked about different elements of the strategy of coping with the offending microbe. Peg, you alluded to effectively a highly targeted strategy, in which you did have lethal intent, but it was a very focused intent around the offending organism. Brad, you talked more about strategies that might avert the need to kill any of the organisms, something more akin to what Stuart was just alluding to. I wonder if you can comment on those strategies, particularly in light of this larger question of what all do we need to do. How important could those strategies be to break through the problem?

DR. RILEY: I confess that my ideas really come from the microbes, themselves. I have spent the last 30 years going out into nature and looking at the interactions between these microbes and seeing how often *they* use a broad-spectrum antibiotic. Not very often. Not many species of bacteria produce them. How often do they use phage? How often do they communicate with small molecules or with bacteriocins? They have worked out a system that survives the ages. The bacteriocins, even when they are used, are still productive. Somehow, they manage to use them in a way that retains their efficacy. That is what allows them to recycle these drugs. It is something we could learn from.

I would also like to add one comment related to Stuart's plurality approach, the one thing we cannot forget is the youngsters that we are teaching and training. That is where the new ideas are going to come from. We run innovation competitions at the University of Massachusetts Amherst, where I am. The things these kids come up with are un-believable. We never would have thought of them and yet they work. I just want us to continue funding research for undergraduates and graduate students, particularly for undergraduates before they become research scientists. That is when the power of the human brain is at its freshest and brightest. We have to support that.

DR. SPELLBERG: I like to go back to first principles before I tackle complex problems. This whole idea of winning the war against microbes? No. We are not going to win a war against organisms that outnumber us by a factor of 10^{22}, outweigh us by 100 million-fold, replicate 500,000 times faster than we do, and have been doing this for 10,000 times longer than our species has existed. What we need to do is, in the immortal words of Dave Gilbert [Professor of Medicine at Oregon Health Sciences University and former president of the Infectious Diseases Society of America], achieve peaceful coexistence. The question is what strategies do we deploy to achieve peaceful coexistence? I think we need to start thinking of infections, by and large, as accidents. There is no advantage in most cases for bacteria to infect us. They are much better off being noninfectious commensals in our gut.

In some cases, we do have to have treatments that remove them from where they are not needed. That may be antibiotics. It may be phage. It may be single-pathogen therapies. It may be immune enhancers. It is all of the above. There isn't going to be a single strategy. We need to relieve the pressure on any one strategy so they can't immediately adapt to that strategy.

I really do think that in the future, we will be increasingly treating infections by a combination of targeted therapies, targeted to the bug and targeted to the host. It is the host's inflammatory response that does cause the majority of signs and symptoms of infections that patients experience.

DR. FINEBERG: Very interesting to think about the microbial world in which we coexist as the natural arrangement. Our job, in a sense, is to figure out how we coexist peacefully, as you put it. It does invert the usual way we think about it, if you will, in the war metaphors of invasion, defense, and destroying the enemy.

No one has talked very much about agriculture and the use of antimicrobials in agriculture, though some of you have alluded to it. Is it just so obviously a foolish thing for us to be doing?

DR. RILEY: Yes.

DR. LEVY: It is. Now, many more people see this as ridiculous. Europe easily eliminated it. We can't do that. We have to go through a legal process, probably go to the legislature, before anything can happen. I have been in this field for 30 years and criticizing these practices. You might say, Levy, you failed because it took 30 years, but it probably would have taken longer if we didn't have this problem of lacking new antibiotics. That just sort of played into it.

Where are antibiotics used? Eighty percent are being given to animals. I was trying to answer this question of multidrug resistance because it can come out of the single use, certainly low dose.

The important point is that the stage is now set. We have to take advantage. We are wasting antibiotics. We are killing our ecology. We are ruining microbiomes. You see a little bit of change. But when you talk to mom and pop farms, which I have done, they only use antibiotics because they think that is what the industry wants. That is the norm. They think that if they don't do it, it is not going to be a product that is equal to the others.

I think there are a lot of negative feelings about this practice. At the time that this was discovered by [Robert] Stokstad and [Thomas] Jukes, they thought they had found the vitamin of the world. He expected a Nobel Prize, Jukes. He said in an interview that he was ready for the Nobel Prize because he found a substitute for feeding people or animals, and because you just have to give them a little bit of an antibiotic. He said it was not working as an antibiotic; it was working like something else. But nobody could ever show how it wasn't working as an antibiotic.

The point is that it had its followers. Now 30 years later, a report in the *New England Journal of Medicine* is published in which researchers are using antibiotics for malnutrition in children in developing countries, in Malawi in this particular case. While they didn't state it, it was the same sort of phenomenon that was being used with the animals. We are giving them antibiotics. We don't know how it works. We don't even know if giving it to them will call the microbiome to become resistant, in which case it won't work anymore. There are so many questions and yet, WHO came out with an edict that said this looks like a good idea. All people should get it. The point of the matter is intelligent people can do unintelligent things.

We did a farm study with 300 chickens that were treated with low-dose tetracycline. The industry that supported this through the Animal Health Institute was shocked when we showed that the antibiotic had an effect on the people working on the farm. They began to excrete resistant bacteria. They thought, "How did that happen? Animals are not sharing the world with us. They are on their own planet." Looking back, there was this naïve belief, really, that there was one world for animals and one world for people.

DR. FINEBERG: I did want to also, if I could, come back to a question, Rima, that your comments made me wonder about. Are we, in our country today, doing enough in surveillance and keeping up to the knowledge of what is happening? How important is this for us, relative to a surveillance global network that will be able to detect problems emerging anywhere? Can you help us understand the state of play there?

DR. KHABBAZ: With regard to surveillance, it varies. Are we doing as best as we can? No. We have limited ability to track certain resistances and certain pathogens. Certainly, we have systems. We are trying to do better, but it is going to need resources to really track resistance as we should across the board.

We have systems. The National Healthcare Safety Network tracks resistance in health care settings. You have something called the Emerging Infections Program that tracks resistance in this community. There are things that we can do to get a more complete, in-depth picture.

DR. LEVY: Surveillance was a nasty word for a long time. The Gates Foundation wouldn't fund anything on surveillance. WHO was very reluctant to get involved with surveillance. Now, all of a sudden, it is the word of the day. WHO has this huge document [2014 report *Antimicrobial Resistance: Global Report on Surveillance*], yet, I can remember clearly being told to remove the word "surveillance." You can use "survey," but you can't use "surveillance." Nobody likes it because they don't think it is worth anything.

DR. KHABBAZ: If you don't want to call it surveillance, that is fine, but if you don't know what you have, you can't deal with a problem. We talked about it here in the United States, but globally, the capacity to find out what resistance they have and be able to track it is very, very weak. One of the points in the Global Health Security Agenda, which is a partnership with other countries, is to improve capacity to detect and prevent and respond. Clearly, antibiotic resistance is a threat. There is an objective to improve the ability to detect antibiotic resistance. It is important. We all breathe the same air and drink the same water and eat the same food.

Antibiotic use in animals, can I say something about that? I want to highlight that FDA is taking steps now. I think everybody might jump in here, but I can't let the opportunity go and not mention that our fellow agency has really taken important steps this year with voluntary label change of antibiotics for animals and limiting the use of antibiotics that are used with humans only for treating infections.

DR. FINEBERG: Thank you very much, Rima. I want to turn in a minute to the audience. You might begin to think if you have questions or comments. We do have a couple of microphones. Brad, I would like to come back to you because of Rima's mention of this idea of partnerships. You made some reference specifically to a new type of public–private partnership that you felt was essential in order to make faster progress. My question to you is why will a partnership between public and private do better than just industry working on it, as we have had? What is it about this problem and the idea that you have of this new partnership that makes it likely to succeed in a way that we can't otherwise?

DR. SPELLBERG: It is a great question. I would say there are two categories of public–private partnerships, and they solve different problems. In the first category, which I will come back to in a second, for-profit industry takes the lead and gets grants or contracts from government to help defray cost and risk.

The second category is a 501(c) nonprofit. It is easier to envision why the nonprofit matters. It is not driven by profit motive. If you are not driven by profit motive, a $50-million-a-year drug or a $10-million-a-year drug is perfectly viable, which would get flushed down the toilet the second it came up in a boardroom in a for-profit company. The nonprofit allows you to select drugs that meet an unmet need, irrespective of market size. That is the importance.

In the first category, the example that GlaxoSmithKline or Achaogen provide is really important. In a large company, revenue—the research and development (R&D) funding stream—actually sets up a competitive relationship between each division in the company. The anti-infective division at GlaxoSmithKline is not competing with Pfizer and Novartis; it is competing with the oncology division and the arthritis division at GlaxoSmithKline.

They have a very limited amount of money that comes to them. How do they stretch those dollars? They go get government grants and contracts so they can develop more than one drug at a time and build a portfolio.

When you look at the net present value (NPV) calculation, which is how most but not all companies determine which drugs are going to be developed, you have to flip it on its head. Revenue is the minority component of the NPV calculation. By far, the biggest driver of NPV is time because of the time cost of money, time discounting. If you can reduce development time and the development dollars are cut in half because half of them are paid for by government, the NPV calculation starts to look much more favorable. In a private for-profit company, if they can tap into R&D dollars from government and decrease upfront costs and shave years off the time line, that will have a profound effect on the ability of that division to develop new drugs.

DR. FINEBERG: Thank you so very much. The floor is open to your questions or comments. Please approach one of the microphones, identify yourself, and address the question to any of the panelists.

DR. PRICE: Lance Price from The George Washington University. It is great to hear this panel of some of my heroes. I have one question and one comment. As far as this new model for developing drugs—private–public partnerships, don't we also need a new model for managing the drugs? It seems the for-profit model of maximizing profit, maximizing sales within a quarter is directly in opposition to what we know about using antibiotics, which is to use as little as possible. If you could comment on that, Dr. Spellberg, I would appreciate it.

DR. SPELLBERG: Yes, I think that is absolutely right. On the one hand, we are actually supposed to have management strategies in place. They just don't work very well. We are supposed to have stewardship programs in place, but we need to make them much more effective, as we have discussed. A big part of moving away from the entrepreneurial model is to have lower upfront costs and the time line for development is faster and you are meeting an unmet need so you can charge a higher price, and if you do, that is a completely different label that the FDA is going to give the drug.

This is not "gorillacilin" that treats every infection. This is a new drug to treat abdominal infections caused by a pan-resistant bacteria. It is a much smaller number of people. You charge more money for each course so the overall market size is still profitable for the company, but you have much less marketing going on. If it is a narrow label, there is less marketing. That, in combination with much more empowered stewardship programs, helps protect use.

DR. PRICE: Just a comment now. We heard about the FDA's progress on this issue of antibiotic use in agriculture. I would say that we should point out that this is a voluntary guidance. It is only addressing growth promotion. We are not even talking about routine disease prevention, preventing diseases that are occurring because of the way we are raising animals, production diseases.

This comes back to surveillance. Without surveillance in place, without monitoring what drugs are being used, in what quantities, for which animals, for what purpose, through which methods, we have no way to see whether these new guidances are successful, whether the industry just switches from growth promotion to routine disease prevention. What I fear is that this is an image of action, when, in fact, we are not doing anything. That allows us to sit back and think that this is okay.

DR. SPELLBERG: I have a much less developed frontal lobe than any of the other panelists. I am just going to tell you point blank there is no scientific debate here about what needs to happen. This is like debating whether global warming is occurring with ExxonMobil. We all know what needs to happen. The issue is how we get the political will to have Congress pass the law. The FDA cannot do what we want them to do without law. Congress will not let them ban growth promotional antibiotics or antibiotics, generally. We need Congress to move on this. That is really where we are at.

DR. FINEBERG: Thank you for both the question and comment.

MS. LITWIN: I am Tamara Litwin. I am a graduate student at the National Heart, Lung, and Blood Institute at NIH. This question is mostly for Dr. Khabbaz, but I am happy for everyone to weigh in. We talked about the U.S. regulatory environment mostly and the European Union, Western Europe, which is very developed. But in some developing countries, antibiotics are available over the counter. People can just go in and self-diagnose and take what they like for as long as they like or as short as they like. How do you think the United States and those countries need to deal with that issue, with the misuse of antibiotics in humans in developing countries, in particular, without overhauling the health care system of the world, which is a bit of a large task?

DR. KHABBAZ: Thank you for the question. It is a hugely important one. As you point out, antibiotics are obtained over the counter. There are so many different systems and approaches—regulatory, social, economic, and cultural—to medicine and treatment, and that makes it a lot more complex. There is no one size fits all solution.

I alluded to the Global Action Plan that WHO is developing. The idea is that there would be many different approaches in different parts of the world. There are also places where people cannot access antibiotics. In some places, you have it sold over the counter and then in others people can't access the right antibiotics needed to treat children that die from respiratory bacteria and infections. How do you decrease the use and, at the same time, make sure antibiotics are available for those who need it? It is complex.

DR. LEVY: I would just say that here is the problem of not having enough professional people in the country to begin with to monitor the drugs. Each country has its own way. The best thing you can do is try to steer them into a stewardship that agrees, in large part, with the rest of the world. That is why the Alliance for Prudent Use of Antibiotics is working at the grassroots level to get each country to develop its own guidelines. It can't be universal. We learned that in 1981 when the Alliance was established. You want to avoid it looking like it is an

American issue and that you are going to correct it. I think it is best handled, and it is being handled, difficult as it is, at the country level.

DR. FINEBERG: Thank you very much.

DR. OVER: My name is Mead Over. I am with the Center for Global Development. I am an economist. Dr. Fineberg, I want to congratulate you on a remarkable panel.

One concept that was never mentioned by any of the speakers was that of fitness. I have done most of my health economics work on HIV, where the impression is that the resistant strains are less fit and that there is a fitness cost. I didn't hear that mentioned. Is this because you were talking about bacteria? I was wondering if you could make some comparative remarks about the danger of fitness in viruses and also, for example, in parasites like the malaria parasite?

The second question has to do with the proportion of the problem that is American. This is related to the climate issue that came up earlier. I think part of the inertia within the U.S. Congress with respect to dealing with the climate issue is that there is this perception that, yes, we are a large part of the problem, but really even a total change of American policy vis-à-vis climate would have almost no effect if we can't get the rest of the world to move with us. Is that also true with respect to the problem we are talking about here today? Is the United States so much of the resistance problem that we could have a really dramatic impact on the global resistance problem by just solving the problem here? If the FDA clamps down on animals, that is going to be a big part of that solution?

DR. RILEY: As an evolutionary biologist, fitness is my currency. That is how we think about how things work. The problem with antibiotic resistance is that I can select for a resistant mutant that makes it so that my *E. coli* can't grow. However, I can go out into nature and find similar mutants that are perfectly happy in the environment, that are present in frequencies of 30 or 40 percent in a population.

The problem is that we tend not to think about what is really affecting the fitness of that bacterial cell. We have no idea what these antibiotic resistance genes actually do for a living. We name them antibiotic resistance genes, but these antibiotic resistance genes are 2 billion years old. Let me say that again like Carl Sagan. Billions of years old.

Clearly, if they evolved for antibiotics, they are in a whole new world right now. They are not doing those jobs anymore or—and this is my own personal prediction—they never did to begin with, but have been co-opted because they did something that helped, for example, pumping an antibiotic out.

We have no way to predict the fitness. Richard Lenski [Hannah Distinguished Professor of Microbial Ecology, Michigan State University] did a great experiment when he was a postdoctoral fellow in Bruce Levin's lab where they took this mutant that they had selected in *E. coli* that was not very fit and they just let it grow in a chemostat. After a couple generations it was more fit than its ancestor.

DR. FINEBERG: Would anyone like to respond to the second question of what proportion of the problem is within the capacity of the United States acting on its own, if it had the will to act, to actually control the problem?

DR. LEVY: There have been multiple studies that have shown both within a single country across geography and transnationally, a very good correlation—it is not 100 percent, nothing in biology is—between the local tonnage of antibiotics dumped into the environment and resistance rates. Information from the European Antimicrobial Resistance Surveillance Network (EARS-Net) is striking. When you compare national antibiotic usage and national antibiotic resistance rates across the EU, it is amazing how they are correlated.

The majority of the problem we face in the United States is homegrown. That is not to say that we don't have imports because we do, but we know that the less we use locally, the less resistance we will have.

DR. FINEBERG: Thank you very much. We have two more questioners. We will take both of those and then we will wrap up and ask for a final comment if anyone would like to make it at that time.

MS. MAHBUB: Hi. My name is Rifaiyat Mahbub. I work on drug resistance at the Center for Global Development. Thanks for such a great panel. All of you had mentioned the use and overuse of antibiotics and that leading to the problem of drug resistance. To me, it seems like it is a classic market failure problem where the true cost of using antibiotics in society is not being reflected in the prices. I was wondering if any of you on the panel could talk about raising the prices of antibiotics and if it is something you considered.

My other question is to Dr. Spellberg. You had talked about implementing pay-for-performance schemes for antibiotic prescriptions. I was wondering if you could elaborate a little bit on that and how you are going to differentiate across diseases and across doctors. I, as a patient, may choose to go to a particular doctor because he is particularly good and I have a particularly invasive disease. How is a pay-for-performance scheme that incentivizes people who prescribe the lowest number of prescriptions different from pharmaceutical companies giving cash incentives out to doctors, which was what led to overprescription? Are we going to enter an era of underprescription? How would pay-for-performance prevent that?

DR. SPELLBERG: Regarding the first question, John Rex [Vice President and Head of Infection, Global Medicines Development, AstraZeneca] and I have published papers, along with Priya Sharma from the London School of Economics, on antibiotic pricing. It is very clear that we price antibiotics ridiculously low relative to their value by any cost-efficacy metric you want to use. You could go to the extreme and look at oncology pricing where you get very little return on investment from many drugs and pay $50,000-$80,000 per course. We are unhappy if we pay $1,000 for a course of antibiotics.

If you look at our *Nature Reviews Drug Discovery* publication, we modeled a novel therapy to treat carbapenem-resistant *Acinetobacter* as an example of a highly resistant Gram-negative. Using standard Medicare performance metrics for cost-efficacy, you could charge $30,000 for a course and still remain well below the $50,000 cost per quality metric that Medicare often uses as a benchmark. We are grossly undercharging for antibiotic use.

If you want to charge more, you have to follow the limited approval mechanisms that we talked about, for example, meet an unmet need and reduce death. If you are just another non-inferiority drug that is the same as everything else, you will never be able to justify that kind of pricing.

Now, to your second question, you are correct. I would say more generally, none of us should be naïve that as we clamp down on inappropriate usage, there are not going to be casualties. I like to tell this example: at an inner city infectious disease conference several years ago now, a sister hospital presented a 28-year-old patient who came to their urgent care clinic with a sore throat, fever, and malaise. They had put in strict protocols. That patient was given no antibiotics and was sent home on chicken soup. She came back 3 days later not feeling any better and they reassured her again and gave her some Tylenol and sent her home. The next week she was diagnosed with Lemierre's disease, which is a blood clot in her jugular vein. She showered emboli all over her body and she died at the age of 28 because she was not given antibiotics. It would have been inappropriate to give her antibiotics. How often does that happen? We don't have great data. The best data would be, say, 1 in 10,000, which is way below the rate of harm that is caused by inappropriate use. Let's not pretend that those 1 in 10,000 events won't happen as we increase appropriate use.

The point of pay-for-performance is to give teeth to the stewardship programs and health care systems that Rima is talking about so they take it seriously and they actually enforce it and drive down inappropriate use. You are right that as a side effect there will be very rare events where harm is caused, but on balance, risk/benefit, clearly more people will be helped by this than harmed by it.

DR. KHABBAZ: I think that is why we need better diagnostics—so that you know what you have and treat for that.

DR. LEVY: Better diagnostics would go a long way in helping us better use antibiotics.

DR. DIXON: [Dennis Dixon, Chief, Bacteriology and Mycology Branch, National Institute of Allergy and Infectious Diseases, NIH] I would like to first start by thanking Harvey and all the panelists. You are all extremely busy people to start with. I know you have gotten a lot busier in the last 6 months or so given the prominence this question has taken on because of the appreciation for the problem.

It was very gratifying to hear that the strategies you all individually mentioned are consistent with what the National Institutes of Health has just published on the Web. If you are interested in reading that—and you may be since you all came to hear this topic—*NIAID's Antibacterial Resistance Program: Current Status and Future Directions, 2014* is available online. It contains an overview of the opportunities we have outlined at the NIH. We put forward seven representative strategies. They included such things as using the microbiome to target and attack the problem; using the host for immune modulation, be it vaccines, be it the innate immune system, or other approaches we don't even know about yet; or using this concept of antivirulence strategies where you disarm, but you don't harm. With this approach, you are not posting a direct selective pressure threat on the pathogen; you are trying to find a way to subdue the problem and then counter with antibacterials.

That is there for your reading. I think you will see beautiful consistency that we hope to be targeting with national funding opportunities and international funding opportunities. We also make the point that you have to put things in context. It is not just drugs; it is also diagnostics and it is prevention, such as in vaccines that can be approached through basic, translational, and clinical research. I will stop there and thank you all once again for your efforts and for taking the time to come here.

DR. FINEBERG: Thank you so much, Dennis, for your comment. Let me just ask if any of the panelists has any final observation you would like to register that we haven't had a chance to elicit from the questions and discussion? Anything anybody likes to add? I know this is not a reticent group so I am going to jump in and seize the moment to say that I know we will all enjoy talking with them much more completely during our reception.

I want to just conclude by suggesting that we have come to grips today with a problem that is urgent, that is ubiquitous, that is long term, and that has many dimensions that simultaneously need to be dealt with if we are going to have any hope of improving our situation, not necessarily even fully resolving the problem. We have, I would submit, near-term challenges around practice today. We have intermediate-term challenges around the adoption and implementation of sounder policies. We have long-term opportunities with the right array of research to come up with the creative solutions that will help improve humanity's balance against and with the microbial world with which we live.

DR. LEVY: Harvey, I won't prolong it much, but I just think that the international/global feature of this problem should not be denied. Even your title, Antimicrobial Resistance: A Problem Without Borders, says that. I think it is important to realize that we aren't alone and there are countries throughout the world that are struggling with this, some worse than we. I think one way we can help is to give them aid.

DR. FINEBERG: Thank you very much for all the observations, for all of your participation, for your questions and comments. Thank you all very much. Please join me in thanking our panelists.

Biosketches

Harvey V. Fineberg, M.D., Ph.D., was President of the Institute of Medicine (IOM) from 2002 to 2014. He served as Provost of Harvard University from 1997 to 2001, following 13 years as Dean of the Harvard School of Public Health. He has devoted most of his academic career to the fields of health care, public health, and decision making at the individual level and for policy. His past research has included health policy development and implementation, assessment of medical technology, evaluation and use of vaccines, and dissemination of medical innovations.

Dr. Fineberg helped found and served as president of the Society for Medical Decision Making and has been a consultant to the World Health Organization. Prior to becoming President of the IOM, he chaired and served on a number of panels at the IOM, including committees on AIDS, new imaging technologies, priorities for vaccine development, and measures of population health. He chairs the board of the Carnegie Endowment for International Peace and is chair-elect of the board of the William and Flora Hewlett Foundation and of the China Medical Board. He also serves on the boards of the Josiah Macy Jr. Foundation and the François-Xavier Bagnoud U.S. Foundation, as well as in a number of advisory capacities, including the National Advisory Committee for the Peterson Institute on Health and the Foresight Committee of the Veolia Environment Institute.

Dr. Fineberg is co-author of the books *Clinical Decision Analysis*, *Innovators in Physician Education*, and *The Epidemic That Never Was*, an analysis of the controversial federal immunization program against swine flu in 1976. He has co-edited several books on such diverse topics as AIDS prevention, vaccine safety, and understanding risk in society.

He has also authored numerous articles published in professional journals.

Dr. Fineberg is a Fellow of the American Academy of Arts and Sciences and the American Association for the Advancement of Science. He is a member of the American Philosophical Society, a Foreign Fellow of the Academy of Athens, a foreign member of the Chinese Academy of Engineering, and a member of the National Academy of Medicine of Mexico.

Dr. Fineberg is the recipient of the Henry G. Friesen International Prize in Health Research, awarded by the Friends of the Canadian Institutes of Health Research; the Innovator in Health Award from NEHI; the Frank A. Calderone Prize in Public Health, awarded by the Mailman School of Public Health, Columbia University; the Stephen Smith Medal for Distinguished Contributions in Public Health from the New York Academy of Medicine; and a number of honorary degrees. He also received the Harvard Medal from the Harvard Alumni Association and the W.E.B. Du Bois Medal, awarded by Harvard's W.E.B. Du Bois Institute for African and African American Research. Dr. Fineberg earned his bachelor's degree, master's degree in public policy, and doctoral degrees from Harvard University.

Rima F. Khabbaz, M.D., is Deputy Director of Infectious Diseases and Director of the Office of Infectious Diseases at the Centers for Disease Control and Prevention (CDC). Prior to her current position, she served as Director of CDC's National Center for Preparedness, Detection, and Control of Infectious Diseases and held other leadership positions across the agency's infectious disease national centers. She is a graduate of the American University of Beirut, Lebanon, where she obtained both her bachelor's degree in science and her medical doctorate degree. She trained in internal medicine and completed a fellowship in infectious diseases at the University of Maryland, Baltimore.

Dr. Khabbaz joined CDC in 1980 as an epidemic intelligence service officer, working in the Hospital Infections Program. She has made major contributions to advance infectious disease prevention, including leadership in defining the epidemiology of non-HIV retroviruses (HTLV-I and -II) in the United States and developing guidance for counseling HTLV-infected persons, establishing national surveillance for hantavirus pulmonary syndrome following the 1993 U.S. outbreak, and developing CDC's blood safety and food safety programs related to viral diseases. She has also played key roles in CDC's responses to outbreaks of new and/or reemerging viral infections, including Nipah, Ebola, West Nile, SARS, and monkeypox, as well as the 2001 anthrax attacks. She is a fellow of the Infectious Diseases Society of America and a member of the American Epidemiologic Society. In addition to her CDC position, she serves as adjunct professor of medicine (infectious diseases) at Emory University. She is a graduate of the National Preparedness Leadership Initiative at Harvard University and of the Public Health Leadership Institute at the University of North Carolina.

Stuart B. Levy, M.D., is Distinguished Professor of Molecular Biology and Microbiology and of Medicine, and the Director of the Center for Adaptation Genetics and Drug Resistance at the Tufts University School of Medicine, in addition to Staff Physician at the Tufts Medical Center. He cofounded and leads the Alliance for the Prudent Use of Antibiotics, an international nonprofit with 65 country chapters and members in more than 100 countries. He is a past President of the American Society for Microbiology (ASM) and cofounder and part-time Chief Scientific Officer of Paratek Pharmaceuticals, Inc. Dr. Levy has published more than 250 papers, as well as 4 edited books and 2 special journal editions on the subject of antibiotic use and resistance. His 1992 book, *The Antibiotic Paradox: How Miracle Drugs Are Destroying the Miracle*, has been cited widely and translated into four languages.

Dr. Levy has received honorary degrees in biology from Wesleyan University (1998) and from Des Moines University (2001). In 2005, colleagues honored him with the ASM book *Frontiers in Antibiotic Resistance: A Tribute to Stuart B. Levy*. He was awarded ASM's 1995 Hoechst-Roussel Award for esteemed research in antimicrobial chemotherapy, the 2011 Hamao Umezawa Memorial Award by the International Society of Chemotherapy, and the 2012 Abbott-ASM Lifetime Achievement Award. He is a Fellow of the American College of Physicians, Infectious Disease Society of America, the American Academy of Microbiology, and the American Association for the Advancement of Science. He was Chairperson of the U.S. Fogarty Center study of "Antibiotic use and resistance worldwide" and helped write the U.S. Office of Technology Assessment report on antibiotic-resistant bacteria. He consults for international and national organizations, including the World Health Organization, National Academy of Sciences, Institute of Medicine, Food and Drug Administration, and the U.S. Environmental Protection Agency.

Margaret A. Riley, Ph.D., is Professor in the Department of Biology at the University of Massachusetts Amherst. She received her Ph.D. at Harvard University in 1991 and joined the faculty at Yale University, where she was granted tenure and remained for 15 years while developing an internationally renowned research program in antimicrobial drug discovery. She has published more than 100 articles and edited 4 books in her research area. Her early studies in microbial ecology and the evolution of antibiotic resistance suggested an alternative to the current paradigm of antibiotic drug discovery, one that recognizes the power of targeted approaches to therapeutic intervention, which result in lower levels of antibiotic resistance and reduced collateral damage to the healthy human microbiome. In 2009, Dr. Riley cofounded a bio-pharmaceutical company, Bacteriotix, whose mission is to provide proof of concept for this new drug development paradigm, with a focus on therapeutic interventions for catheter-acquired urinary tract infections. In 2009, she cofounded the Institute for Drug Resistance, whose mission is to facilitate novel, multidisciplinary approaches to addressing the challenge of drug resistance, and created a new Gordon Research Conference on Drug Resistance.

In 2008, Dr. Riley created the Massachusetts Academy of Sciences, a nonprofit organization whose mission is to increase levels of civic science literacy. She currently serves as its President and oversees science outreach and education reform efforts aimed at engaging middle and high school students in independent research experiences and providing their teachers with professional development opportunities in inquiry-based teaching methods. She is a fellow of the American Academy of Microbiology and recently joined the Board on Life Sciences of the National Academy of Sciences.

Brad Spellberg, M.D., is Associate Medical Director for Inpatient Services and Associate Program Director for the Internal Medicine Residency Training Program at Harbor-UCLA Medical Center. He is also a Professor of Medicine at the David Geffen School of Medicine at UCLA (University of California, Los Angeles). He received his B.A. in Molecular Cell Biology-Immunology from UC Berkeley. He attended medical school at UCLA and completed his residency in internal medicine and fellowship in infectious diseases at Harbor-UCLA Medical Center. Dr. Spellberg has extensive patient care and teaching activities, including oversight of inpatient care hospitalwide at Harbor-UCLA Medical Center. His research interests range from basic immunology and vaccinology to pure clinical research and outcomes research. His laboratory research has focused on developing a vaccine that targets the bacterium *Staphylococcus aureus* and the fungus *Candida*; the vaccine is undergoing clinical development. Dr. Spellberg is currently working on the immunology, vaccinology, and host defense against highly resistant Gram-negative bacilli, including *Acinetobacter* and carbapenem-resistant Enterobacteriaceae infections.

Dr. Spellberg has worked extensively with the Infectious Diseases Society of America (IDSA) to attempt to bring attention to the problems of increasing drug resistance and decreasing new antibiotics. His research regarding new drug development was a cornerstone of the IDSA's white paper, *Bad Bugs, No Drugs*. As a member and then co-chair of the IDSA's Antimicrobial Availability Task Force, he first-authored numerous IDSA position papers and review articles relating to public policy of antibiotic resistance and antibiotic development. Dr. Spellberg is the author of *Rising Plague*, which he wrote to inform and educate the public about the crisis in antibiotic-resistant infections and lack of antibiotic development.